BID ADIEU TO
STRESS

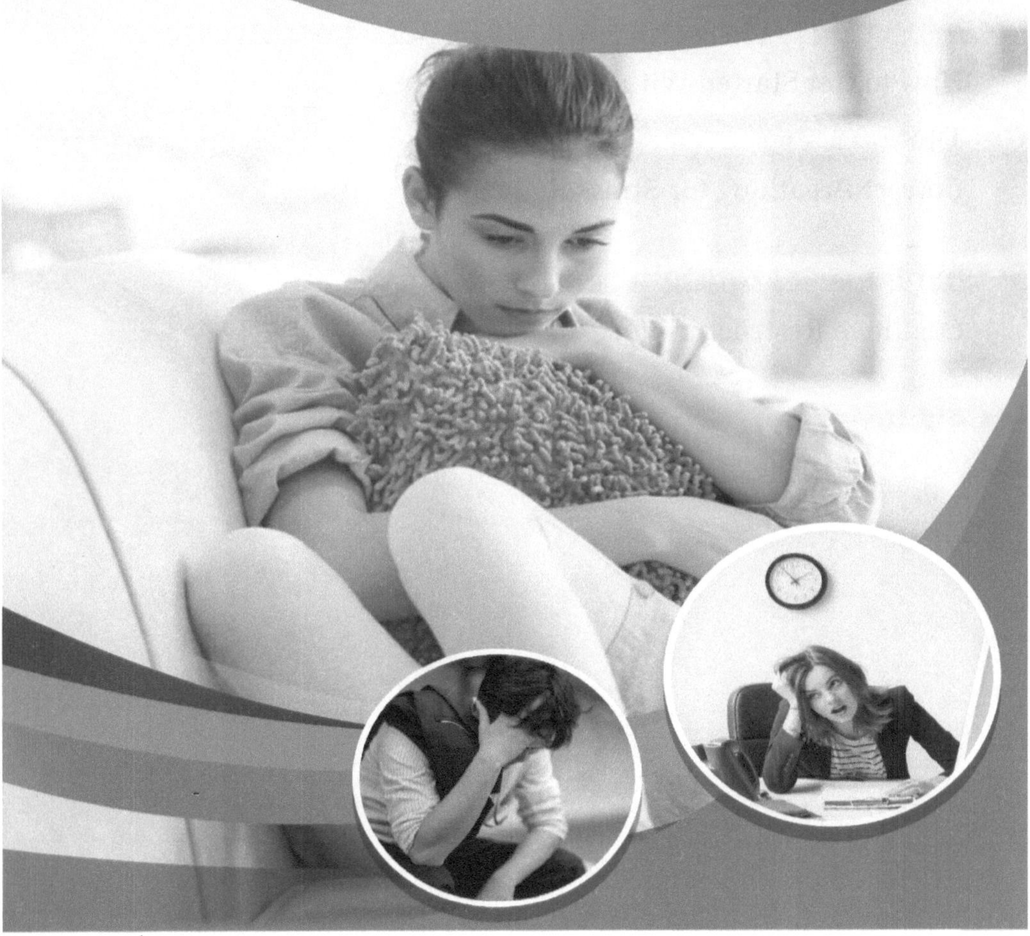

Table of Contents

Chapter 01 - What is Stress and How Does it Damage You?

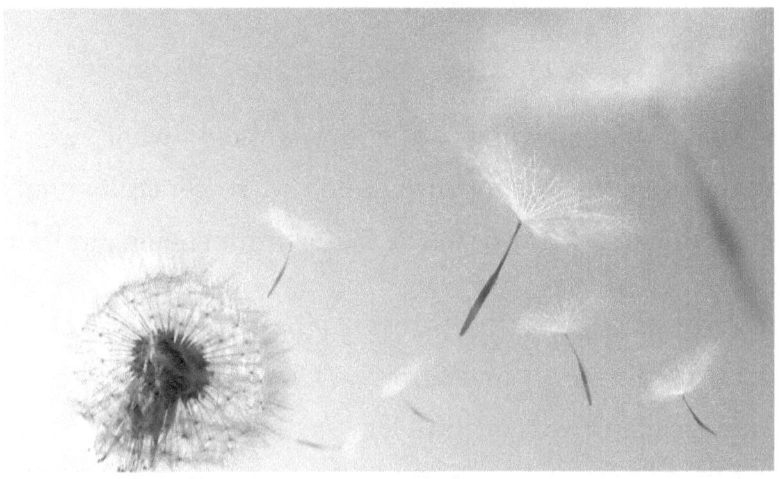

We all know that stress is bad for us and this is something we get told very often. However, it's all too easy to write this off as being a minor nuisance or frustration rather than anything to really worry about. We all get stressed from time to time, right?

In reality though, this is the wrong way to think about stress. While it is fairly common place, that is not to say that it isn't serious. In fact, stress is *incredibly* serious and can cause severe problems both in the short term and long term.

Stress can shorten your lifespan. Ruin your enjoyment. Cause serious illness. Shrink your brain. Hurt your performance. Ruin your relationships. Cause impotence.

Do those sound like small matters?

To understand this better, it can help to look more closely at what precisely stress is. *How* it causes the problems it does and how and why you need to do everything you can to prevent and reduce it.

So What Exactly is Stress?

Stress is what we feel when we're overworked, when we're dreading something that's about to happen or when we're generally unable to relax and stay calm due to outside or inside factors influencing our thoughts.

But it actually goes beyond this. Stress is a basic physiological reaction that is designed to help us focus and survive. In itself it is not a bad thing and is actually rather adaptive. The problem is that it has been taken out of context, which means the positive effects become outweighed by the negative.

Essentially, stress is what causes the 'fight or flight response'. This is a physiological response to perceived danger, designed to improve our chances of survival. If you were to see a lion for example, this would trigger a cascade of effects collectively resulting in the stress response.

This begins when we observe danger or experience fear. Increased activity in our brain, causes the release of adrenaline, as well as dopamine, norepinephrine and cortisol – our stress hormones. These then trigger a number of physiological changes: increasing our heartrate, making us breathe more quickly and making us more acutely focussed on the potential threat.

A list of the symptoms should include:

- Increased heartrate
- Rapid, shallow breathing

- Muscle contraction
- Tunnel vision
- Heightened sensitivity
- Increased blood viscosity
- Suppression of the pain response
- Suppression of the immune system
- Suppression of the digestive system
- Dilation of the pupils
- Dilation of the blood vessels
- Reduction in prefrontal cortex activity (temporo-hypofrontality)

In the short term, this is good for us. In the short term, these things help us to evade danger and win combative situations. Increased muscle tension makes us stronger. Increased blood viscosity makes our blood more likely to clot in case of an injury. Dilated pupils let more light in to improve our vision. Suppression of secondary functions means that more blood can be sent to the muscles and the brain. Reduced pain means we can carry on fighting or running despite injury.

In short, anything that can help you to survive is prioritized, while secondary functions are suppressed. The idea is that once we get to safety, we can then turn off this fight or flight response and instead enter the 'rest and digest' state in order to recover. Once the predator is gone, we can recover.

But the problem is that in our modern environments, predators aren't the main problem. It's rare these days for us to be chased, to get into a fight or to need to escape a forest fire.

What's *not* so rare, is for our boss to shout at us and to tell us that we're late for our deadline. It's not rare for us to be in debt. It's not rare for us to have marital problems.

And unfortunately, the brain interprets all these signals in just the same way: as threats. And this causes the same fight or flight response. But because these types of threats aren't so easily resolved, this means we'll often end up on heightened alert for a longer period of time.

This is also why stress causes impotence in men. If you are highly stressed, blood is sent *everywhere* except the genitals!

And this takes a tremendous toll on our bodies.

As you might imagine: it is not good for you when your immune system and digestive system are suppressed for days. It's also not good for your brain to be flooded with norepinephrine and cortisol. It's not good for your heartrate to stay elevated, or your blood pressure to stay high.

This is the problem with *chronic* stress as opposed to acute stress. And it's the problem with heightened levels of stress, as opposed to the gentle, motivating force of 'eustress'. We'll look at all of this more in the long term, but suffice to say that the longer stress like this continues, the more you start to feel drained, malnourished, fatigued, ill and possibly eventually depressed.

How Stress Damages the Brain

When we are stressed, it effectively makes us less intelligent. This is due to the reduction in pre-frontal activity, which in turn is designed to make us more focussed and alert. Essentially, the pre-frontal cortex is the part of the brain responsible for forward planning, creative thinking and other 'high-order' brain activity.

When you are being chased by a lion though, it is really not the time to be thinking about the meaning of life!

So shutting down this part of the brain and placing your focus on feedback from your senses makes much more sense.

Of course that's not particularly useful in the workplace though: and this is why the stress response is so seriously *un*helpful when we have to give a presentation, answer a question on the spot or go on a date. This is when we lose all articulation and start stammering and saying useless things.

Slightly longer-term is adrenal fatigue. This is what happens when your brain has exhausted its supply of adrenaline and other stress hormones. That might sound like a good thing but you actually need a little norepinephrine, dopamine and cortisol to stay motivated – and even to wake up in the morning! Adrenal fatigue leaves you listless, demotivated and potentially depressed. It can also cause what is known as 'learned helplessness' – a condition where you essentially completely give up because your brain has been conditioned to learn that any attempts to change its situation will be met with failure. Not good!

Worse, when you are highly stressed, it can lead to *long term* problems for your brain health. As we briefly mentioned: it can *literally* shrink your brain! Studies show that in the long term, it leads to structural changes that shrink the hippocampus and shrink grey matter – the all-important neural connections throughout the brain. Even a single, severe traumatic event can result in significant reductions in the medial PFC, anterior cingulate and subgenual regions of the brain. The effects of 'cumulative adversity' meanwhile, cause smaller volumes in the medial prefrontal cortex (the PFC), insular cortex and anterior cingulate regions.

These regions of the brain correspond with emotional control, decision-making, reasoning and self control.

In other words, the eventual result of stress is to leave you more reactionary, more depressive, more impulsive and less disciplined.

From here, *every* aspect of your life will start to see negative effects. But there are things you can do about it...

Chapter 02 – The Complexity of Your Stress Systems

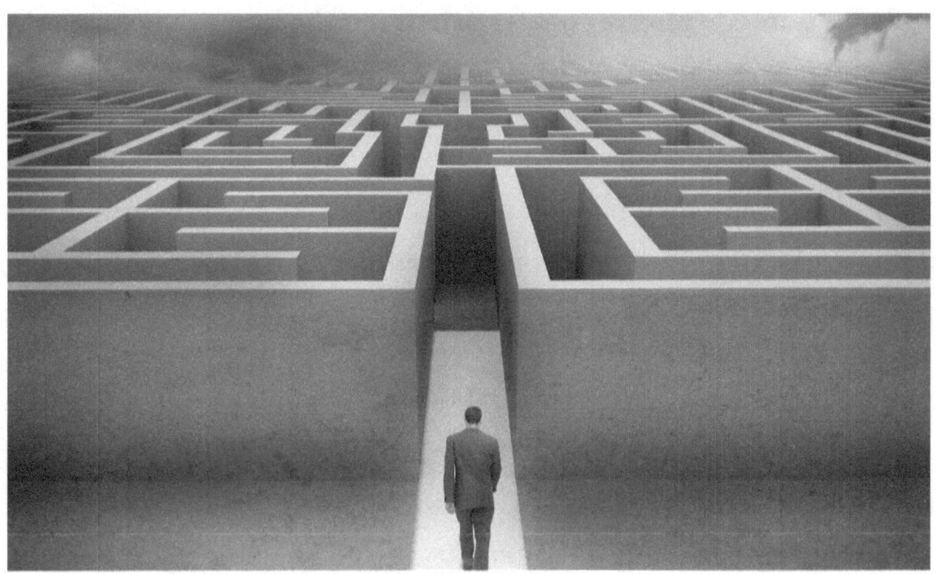

But what if you're not stressed?

What if your work isn't particularly high pressured, your relationships are good and you have plenty of money? Does that mean you're fine?

Probably not. Unfortunately, many other aspects of our modern lifestyles cause symptoms similar to those of stress.

One example is our use of technology and artificial lighting. The brain is designed to use external cues ('zeitgebers' to use correct terminology) to set its own biological rhythms including the sleep-wake cycle (circadian rhythm).

This actually triggers the release of stress hormones at certain times of day. That's because stress hormones are one of the tools that the body uses to wake itself up when you are sleeping. The release of stress hormones like cortisol and norepinephrine triggers activity in the brain that stirs you out of sleep and makes you fully alert.

But if the light is on at night, or you're looking at your phone in the evening, this will cause the release of similar stress hormones right when you're meant to be relaxing. That means you'll continue to feel alert and won't give your brain time to recover.

And what doesn't help is the way that everything on the web and on TV is designed to grab our attention and pull us this way and that – this has been shown to cause effects similar to ADHD in the long term and make it harder for us to concentrate on any one thing for very long.

How Physiological Changes Trigger Stress

The above is an example of how stress is entirely a result of what's going on in your life or even of what you're thinking. Instead, stress can be a result of outside factors that physically influence you.

A way to think of it is like this:

Physical Sensations > Feelings > Emotions > Thoughts > Behaviors

That is to say that your emotions are very often the result of *physical* things affecting your physiology.

For example, if you're in a colder environment, this actually increases the amount of cortisol and the amount of norepinephrine. Physiologically, this is the same as low-level stress and that's why a cold shower is a great way to wake yourself up!

This is also why being cold for too long can make you ill – as the stress response is suppressing your immune system.

Likewise, if you are hungry, then this triggers a physiological type of stress. Essentially, hunger causes your brain to release cortisol due to a decrease in blood sugar. When blood sugar is low, cortisol is released and the body responds to this as it would any other type of stress.

Why? Because as far as the body is concerned, this *is* a form of danger. If you are hungry, then you need to become active and get out there in order to seek out a source of food. Ghrelin, the hunger hormone, is released alongside cortisol and myostatin which breaks down tissue to provide energy.

When you eat on the other hand, this causes a sudden spike in your blood sugar. That in turn will cause you to release insulin, which absorbs the sugar for use around the body (either in the muscles and brain, or to be stored as fat).

This also has the effect of leaving behind another substance called 'tryptophan', which is found in most foods but doesn't get absorbed. Tryptophan makes its way through the circulatory system all the way to the brain, where it crosses the blood brain barrier and converts to serotonin (as it is a 'precursor' to serotonin). Serotonin is the 'feel good hormone' and it's also a precursor itself: this time to melatonin – the sleep hormone.

This is why when you eat a large meal, you tend to feel full, then happy, then sleepy. Christmas dinner ring any bells?

This is the opposite of the stress response. This is the aforementioned 'rest and digest' response.

And this is another cycle that your body goes through constantly: it moves from fight or flight, to rest and digest. You just don't notice this because in a perfect world, that shift will be subtle and you won't feel it too much. You just move slightly up and down the spectrum, becoming slightly *more* alert and focussed and then slightly *less* so.

Nevertheless though, this constant fluctuation *does* have an impact on things like your productivity and your mood. And it is also closely tied to the sleep-wake cycle. When you wake up for instance, you are in a fasted state having slept all night: thus you have high cortisol.

Chapter 03 - Ways to Manage Normal Stress

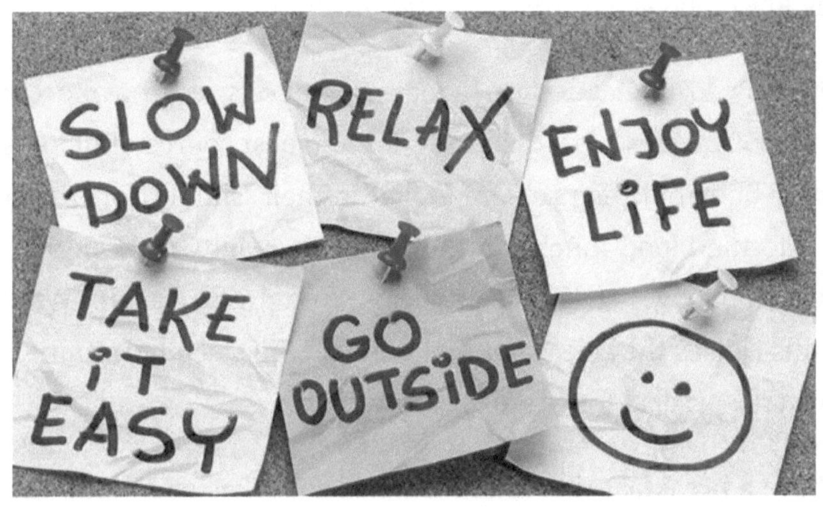

Just understanding these factors, you can hopefully see that stress isn't a 'bad thing' necessarily: rather it is a useful and required part of a normal, healthy, functioning body. In fact, as we've discussed, a little stress is necessary in order to help you feel more alert, more focussed and more productive. If we never had even a small amount of stress hormones in our system, then we would spend all our time highly rested and too laid back to get any actual work done!

The key is to make sure that those stress levels stay at this optimal level, as well as to try and get your natural cycles to line up with the times when you need to be most productive during the day.

And we can start by hijacking some of the physiological aspects we've already discussed...

Managing Blood Sugar

One very simple way to keep your stress at bay, is to avoid letting your blood sugar drop too low. We've already seen that low blood sugar triggers the release of cortisol and other stress hormones and so it follows that by avoiding low blood sugar, we can avoid this fate.

The best way to manage your blood sugar levels, is to avoid consuming simple carbohydrates. Carbohydrates are the best source of blood sugar for the human body but the problem is that in their 'simple' form, they release energy into the blood much too quickly. This results in a sudden spike in sugar, which then gets taken up and leaves you drained again. What's more, is that this causes the release of melatonin – the sleep hormone – as we've seen earlier. Not ideal for working.

If you have a breakfast that is made up of pancakes and syrup then, it will wake you up and make you feel good in the morning but an hour later you'll start to run low on energy and that will cue the release of cortisol.

So instead, try consuming a source of calories that will release the sugar more gradually into your bloodstream. A great choice is some form of complex carbohydrate, such as oats. This takes longer to reach the blood stream, providing a steady stream of blood sugar and preventing you from going into alert 'starvation' mode.

Conversely, fat will also have the same effect. When you consume a saturated fat, this will once again sit in the stomach while it gets broken down, providing you with a steady release of energy that will help you go about your business throughout the day.

Stay Comfortable

Comfort is fantastic for reducing stress and this has been shown in studies to help boost creativity. It only takes your keys to be digging into your pocket for example, for your body to consider you as uncomfortable and potentially being damaged. Thus, you will find that if you can sit in a more supportive and comfortable chair and also ensure the temperature is right and you are surrounded by things that put you at ease (plants have been shown to do this well for most people), then you will start to feel a lot calmer – even when you're at work and other stresses are being thrown at you.

Spend Time Away From Screens

Computers, smartphones and television are all great. They're entertaining and they're great for productivity. Unfortunately though, they're also very bad for us when it comes to stress hormones. We've already discussed how light from screens can trigger the release of cortisol and we've seen that the constant messages and alerts essentially trigger a series of small stress responses while we're surfing the web.

This is manageable but it becomes problematic when you spend too much time on the computer. Simply going for occasional walks and taking breaks from the screen throughout the day then will be a great way to help your body recover.

Another tip is to take time off just before bed. If you aim to have a restorative and restful night's sleep, then you need to give yourself time to 'wind down' just before you hit the sack. Taking time away from computers is one of the best ways to do this, so why not have a bath before bed with some candles instead? Or read by a more natural type of light? Give yourself half an hour of 'screen off' time and you'll find you get to sleep much quicker and feel more restored in the morning.

No can do? If you absolutely can't separate yourself from your gadgets at the end of the day, then try using software that will reduce the amount of 'blue light' coming from the screen. Redshift technology will help you block the most damaging wavelengths from your devices and thereby create a more restful light. An alternative is to wear 'blue blocking shades' which can block all blue light in your environment before bed!

Get Rid of Your Alarm

You know what really isn't helping your stress levels?

Your morning alarm!

The reason alarms tend to choose from a generic range of sounds, is that bleeps and ringing sounds are unnatural. These sounds don't occur in nature and thus we are attuned to them and they make us naturally sit up and take notice. In other words: they trigger a stress response.

And now bear in mind that when this happens, you are often in the very deepest stage of sleep. What a way to start your day! Rudely woken from the depths of sleep by a blaring noise, only to find yourself in a pitch dark room.

There are two much healthier alternatives to consider...

Fitness Tracker

One option is to use a fitness tracker/smart watch that has a smart alarm function. These work by monitoring your heartrate and your movement during the night, in order to estimate how awake or asleep you are at any given stage. Using this information, they can then wake you up at the point when you're in light REM sleep, rather than deep SWS sleep. The result is that you're woken at a point when you're already coming around anyway –

and this is combined with a gentle nudge from a vibration, rather than a loud ringing.

Daylight Lamp

Better yet, is to use a daylight lamp. These are lamps that are designed to create a wavelength similar to that of the sun – with plenty of blue light! In that way, these are the opposite of redshift technology or blue blocking shades.

These lights will then be built into alarm, that are able to gradually get brighter as it nears the point that you set to wake up at. This helps to gradually stir you into wakefulness, by mimicking the effects of a sunrise. You start to feel more and more awake and your brain produces hormones associated with waking up – such as cortisol and nitric oxide.

While this is a stress response, it's a much milder and more natural stress response to the one that is caused by the sudden blaring of an alarm. The result is that you feel calmer and happier during the day and that you'll be better able to sustain levels of activity later thanks to a more accurate body clock.

Rethink Your Commute

Commuting to work is one of the worst things you can do for your stress levels throughout the day.

Did you know for example, that a typical commute will trigger huge amounts of what is considered to be the only 'universal fear'?

So what is this universal fear? It's things moving quickly toward you. Across all cultures and all demographics, moving something quickly towards a person's face will cause them to recoil and to see an increase in their heartrate and their stress response. Now think about a typical commute – filled with people moving rapidly towards you, lots of noise, lots of pollution and generally huge amounts of chaos. Before your day has even begun, you'll be experiencing huge amounts of stress.

This might be outside of your control. But if it *is* within your control, then make sure you do anything you can to avoid this kind of commute. Even just going in an hour earlier to avoid the rush-hour may be a good choice.

Rethink Your Morning Coffee

You know what else *really* isn't helping your stress in the morning?

That cup of coffee!

When you drink coffee, you are essentially experiencing the stress response in a cup. That's because coffee works by triggering something akin to a stress response.

It starts by mimicking a molecule we all have in our brains called 'adenosine'. Adenosine is a by-product of the energy systems in the body and it builds up over time as we are active. The more you use your brain power, the more of this substance accumulates.

The problem, is that adenosine is also an inhibitory neurotransmitter. The more adenosine builds up, the tireder we get and the less active the brain becomes. This is one of the reasons that we find ourselves feeling tireder and less cognitive able as the day drags on.

Drink caffeine though and the brain's 'adenosine receptors' get confused. They absorb caffeine instead of adenosine and this means the adenosine has nowhere to go and can't work. This in turn, gives you an instant boost in energy levels by making you feel more awake and focussed.

This also leads to a general increase in brain activity though and this is where the stress response comes in. The brain notices this sudden wakefulness and what do you know, it assumes that something very important must be going on. Thus, we see a release of more neurotransmitters associated with stress! Our good friends cortisol, norepinephrine, adrenaline and dopamine. This increases the heartrate, dilates the pupils, suppresses the immune system... all the things that any other stress response does.

Caffeine in itself is not bad. In small doses it can help boost memory and wakefulness and it's actually protective against all kinds of neurodegenerative diseases in the long term. But what it also is, is a quick way to make any stressful situation worse. If you've got a busy day, you just commuted during rush hour and you sit down at work to drink a big cup of coffee, you're only going to make yourself *more* stressed and wired.

And guess what? Once again, this is going to result in a crash shortly afterward when your energy levels have been depleted.

Don't drink caffeine as part of a routine. Drink it when you need that extra push – don't rely on it and don't combine it with other stress.

Chapter 04 - How Does Meditation Reduce Stress?

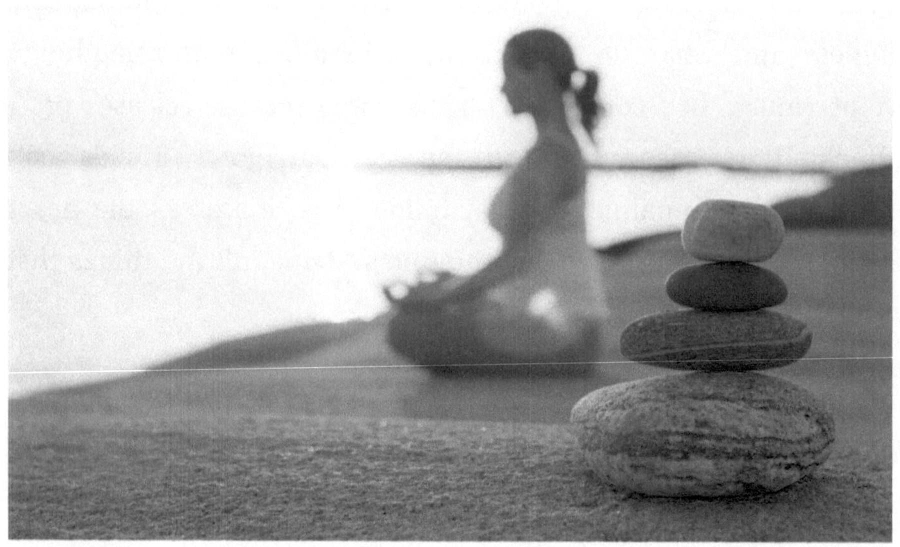

While all these changes can help, there is one thing that is more powerful than any other tool when it comes to combating stress: meditation.

Meditation is something a lot of people don't fully understand. There is the assumption among some that meditation is somehow 'mystical' or that it is necessarily linked with religion. Neither of these things is true.

There are many different types of meditation from transcendental, to mindfulness, to religious meditation but all of them really just have one thing in common: they involve the purposeful direction of attention inward.

Whether it is reflecting on your own thoughts, praying or just sitting silently and trying to clear your mind, meditation involves making the conscious decision to take control of what you're thinking and to try and stop your thoughts from jumping around everywhere. And when you do this, you will find it has a truly profound effect on your ability to stay calm in stressful situations, to control the nature of your thoughts and to combat many of the negative effects of stress.

In fact, studies show us that meditation can improve the areas of your brain that stress destroys – actually increasing the amount of grey matter in the brain and the amount of whole-brain connectivity. Furthermore, it can help to improve areas of the brain specifically related to motivation, attention and willpower. One study shows that it only takes 8 weeks to see amazing positive changes to the brain and restoration of grey matter in particular.

People who use meditation will usually report that they feel generally calmer, happier and more at peace throughout the day. This results in a better mood, heightened attention and general improvements in cognitive function and productivity.

All these things mean that meditation is actually the perfect antidote to stress and can undo a lot of the damage that meditation causes. Apart from anything else, meditation will help you to take a small break from the constant stress of daily life and from the racing thoughts that come with this. More to the point though, it will teach you to take control of racing thoughts at will and simply to put them to one side.

Meanwhile, allowing your brain some time to enjoy this highly relaxed state will encourage the reparation of neurons and the cementing of things you've learned through the day.

Finally, it makes sense that areas controlling self-control would develop during the process of meditation. Meditation uses certain brain areas and we now know that the more you use an area of the brain, the more it grows.

This works just like using a muscle and is a process known as 'brain plasticity'.

And by practicing reflecting on your own mental state and being more aware of your own emotions, it only follows that you would better be able to control it and to avoid letting stress or impulse get the better of you in future.

How to Get Started With Meditation

So this is what meditation does for you and why it is the ideal antidote to stress.

The next question is how can you get started with meditation? Do you need to attend a class? Do you need to be a Buddhist monk?

Fortunately, meditation is actually pretty simple and this is what ends up making it hard even in some cases. A lot of people who first try meditation feel that it is *too* simple and thus assume they must be doing something wrong!

The easiest way to get started if you're a complete beginner, is to try guided meditation. Guided meditation means using a pre-recorded script that will talk you through everything you need to be doing at any given stage. Essentially, this works to help direct your attention and show you what you need to be reflecting on or paying attention to at any given time.

A good one to try is 'Headspace'. This is available as a website and as an app and in either case, you'll find a selection of guided meditations to walk you through. The only downside is that headspace is not free and that after the first 10 sessions, you'll have to start paying.

Fortunately, those first ten sessions are more than enough to give you a taste of meditation and to teach you the basics. From here, you'll then be able to take what you learned and re-apply it in order to continue on your own.

If you'd rather not start a paid system though, then you can always use one of the *many* free YouTube videos that will do the same thing!

In general, most guided meditation will take you through the following steps.

To start with, you will sit somewhere comfortable and close your eyes. Set a timer for 10 minutes, or however long you have until you need to be doing other things. While you should be comfortable, you shouldn't be too reclined or generally put yourself in danger of falling asleep!

The next thing to do, is to bring your attention to the sounds and the world around you. This means just listening to the sounds and noticing what you can hear. This is an interesting exercise in and of itself: if you actually stop to listen you'll be able to pick up on a *lot* more information than you were probably previously aware of.

Don't strain to listen but instead just let the sounds come to you – whether those be barks from dogs next door, the sound of birds or perhaps chatter from someone in another building that you can hear through the walls.

After you have done this for a little while, the next step is to bring your attention in to yourself and to notice how your body feels. This means noticing the way that your weight is distributed on your buttocks. Is it evenly distributed? Are you leaning slightly to one side? Likewise, try to notice the air against your skin, the temperature, any aches and pains etc.

You can then try the 'body scan'. This is something that some people use as the main basis for their meditation and it involves focussing on each part of your own body, starting right from the head and then moving down the body slowly from the face, to the chest, to the legs, to the feet. Each time you get to a point on your body, make a conscious effort to release any tension you might be holding there and to relax.

You can even turn your attention inward further by seeing if you can feel the beating of your own heart, or the movement of your diaphragm.

Either way, we're now going to focus on breathing. This is something that a lot of people will again use as the entire basis of their meditation. Simply count the breaths in and the breaths out and each time you get to ten, start again. The aim now is to have all of your focus and all of your attention on the breathing and not to be distracted by anything outside.
Now, from time to time, you will notice that your thoughts start to drift and that you end up thinking about other things. This is a fantastic example of just how hard we find it to focus on any one thing for a given period of time. It's a fantastic example of just why you *need* this meditation!

Don't fret when it happens though. This is the worst thing you can do! Instead, simply 'notice' that your mind has wandered and then bring your attention *back* to your breathing again. Each time it drifts off, just re-center and don't worry about it.

Focussing on the breathing is simply giving us a way to center our thoughts and to remove the distractions that normally interrupt. This could just as easily work by focussing on anything else: for example, some people will focus on a single word called a 'mantra'. A mantra is what is often used in transcendental meditation for instance and might mean just repeating the word 'Om' in order to busy your internal monologue.

Finally, the last stage of our guided meditation is going to be to just let the thoughts wander freely and to let them go wherever they want to.

This last stage is essentially mindfulness meditation. The idea is that you're going to detach yourself from those thoughts and simply 'watch them' rather than feeling emotionally affected by them.

This last part is the part where you get to really relax and stop 'fighting' your brain and it's a great way to end. Then bring your focus back to your breathing, then back to your body, back to the world around you and eventually open your eyes.

Congratulations, that was your first meditation session!

Tips

Learning to meditate and making it a part of your life are two very different things and a lot of people reading this are now going to struggle to adopt this new behavior in a meaningful way.

The first issue is that a lot of people get frustrated when they feel that their meditation isn't 'working' and they thus give up. This is entirely the wrong way to look at meditation – this is not a means to an end but rather a relaxing place you can come and visit whenever you need it, or a great interlude before you start your day.

This extends to how you start out. A lot of people want things to go perfectly right away and they'll wonder why they haven't achieved enlightenment as soon as they close their eyes! Then their hair gets in their face, they become stressed that they aren't doing it right and they get up. Then they need to itch. Then they're not comfortable.

Don't worry about it. It's fine to move. It's fine to open your eyes for a moment. All that's important is that you then bring your attention *back*. In time, you'll find you are less distracted. But to begin with, you won't be ready for that yet and you mustn't get frustrated when you find that distractions do arise.

The next tip is to think carefully about how you're going to sustain your meditation training and make it a feasible part of your routine. A lot of resources will tell you how easy it should be to take 10 minutes out of your day. They'll claim that 'everyone' has five minutes.

In reality though, it's *not* easy. If it were, then everyone would already be doing it! Most of us are so busy that we legitimately struggle to find five minutes of free time and so we need to be realistic about what we can and can't achieve.

Look at it this way: it's much better to practice for two minutes twice a week and actually *stick with it*, than it is to try and practice for an hour a day and to give up after day two.

The best thing to do is to find an opportunity when you waste time in the morning or the evening. This might be while your partner goes through the shower in the morning, or it might be when you get home from work. Whatever it is, most of us have a few short periods of time in our usual routine and the great thing about meditation is that you can do it anywhere and with no props. Even if it's on the train to work, or if it is when you get into work 10 minutes early. If you can find a 'slot' that already exists, you'll find it's much easier to fit meditation in and to stick with.

Correct Breathing for Stress Reduction

When meditating it is important to try to remember to breathe properly. And better yet is to try and make this into a habit so that your breathing is better during your waking day as well.

The thing is: a lot of people don't know *how* to breathe well and are unintentionally breathing incorrectly most of the time. Theory has it that the reason for this is closely linked to the way we sit at work.

This is a big deal if you're trying to reduce stress, seeing as your stress levels are closely related to the way you breathe. We've already seen that there is a strong connection between physiology, feelings, emotions and psychology. When we are stressed, we breathe more quickly and not as deeply. But likewise, when we breathe more quickly and not as deeply, we *become* more stressed.

Right now, take both hands and place one on your stomach and one on your chest. Now breathe normally. Which hand is moving first? Is it the hand on your chest or the hand on your stomach?

For most people, the answer is the chest. But to be optimally healthy, it should be the stomach. When we're infants this is how we breathe and it's also how animals breathe. Years of sitting in an office desk though, or on a sofa, mean that we've spent too long with our stomachs compressed and learned to breathe differently.

Stomach breathing means that you are relaxing your abdominal muscles, thereby opening up your abdominal cavity and allowing your diaphragm to drop down into that space. This then creates more room for the lungs and they will automatically inflate as they enlarge. You *then* bring your chest in and open that up to take in even more oxygen and as a result, you breathe a lot more deeply. This oxygenates your body and it calms your heartrate and helps you to feel less stressed.

In fact, one of the very best ways to help yourself feel instantly less stressed, is to start taking deep, controlled breaths. This puts you in a rest and digest state and stops the fight or flight response in its tracks. So if you're about to go to an interview or give a presentation, practicing some controlled breathing for a while is the perfect antidote to the stress you're probably experiencing.

Chapter 05 - Mindfulness and CBT

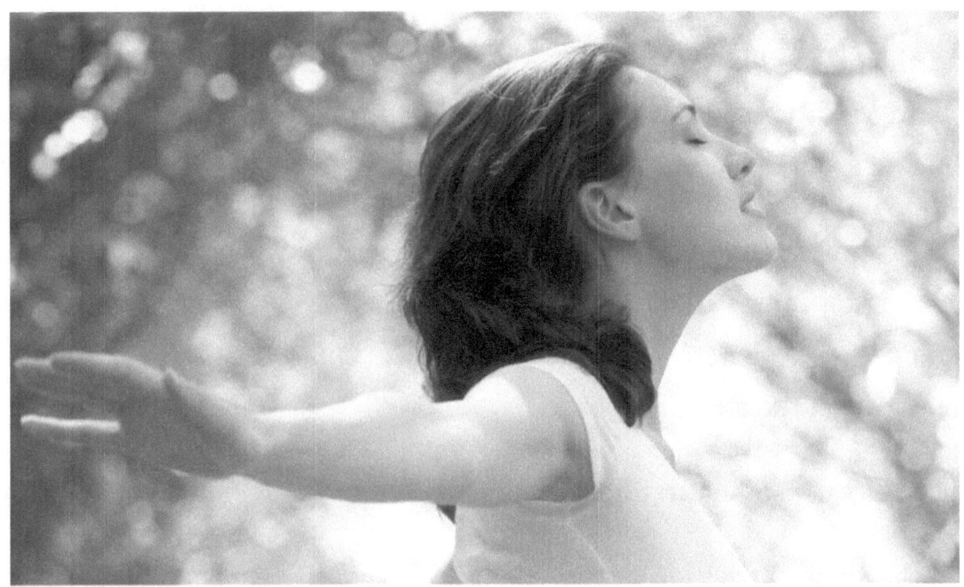

Meditation is not only a fantastic tool, it's also great way to practice being more aware of your own thoughts and feelings, such that you can then take full control of them.

This brings us to the concept of CBT – or cognitive behavioral therapy. CBT is essentially a type of psychotherapeutic intervention that teaches people who struggle with anxiety or other issues, how to better control the nature of their own thoughts.

This all starts with perception, and this is where you can use mindfulness. Remember the part of the meditation we discussed where we mentioned that you should 'watch' the contents of your
thoughts? Try doing this the next time you're stressed: what are you actually thinking?

What you'll find is that when you're stressed, you are imagining the worst and this is what is causing you to get worked up.

And this is the big secret to stress: other than the physiological response that we've discussed, stress is really a result of your *perception* of what's going on around you.

Put it this way: if you're faced with a lion you will get a stress response as soon as you notice it. But if you *believe* the lion is your friend, then you won't get the same stress response. Or if you *think* the lion is a hologram, you won't get the stress response.

The reality doesn't matter here: what matters here is what you are thinking.

And the same is true for all those sources of chronic stress we've discussed so far. If you are struggling with debt and with work, then your perception is that there's a great big lion ahead of you. But if you can convince yourself that there's no benefit to being stressed and if you can convince yourself that it's not worth getting worked up, then you can overcome that stress and your response will be the same as if there was *no* pressure in your life.

Cognitive Restructuring

So how do you do this?

The first step is to note the thoughts that are making you more worked up. If you're stressed about talking in public, then perhaps you are filled with thoughts like:

- What happens if I stutter?
- People are going to laugh at me
- I won't be able to talk

- I don't know my script

None of this is helpful – it makes that lion seem bigger!

You want to replace these for more positive thoughts but simply *telling* yourself it's all alright won't work. You need to genuinely believe it.

To do this, you use cognitive restructuring. A big part of this is 'thought challenging', where you challenge your assumptions and test just how accurate they're likely to be.

Are you really likely to stutter? Do you normally stutter?

Would people really laugh at you? Are the people in your audience that rude and unkind? And if they do laugh at you – why does it matter? You won't have to see them again. Everyone knows that people stutter from time to time. And a little embarrassment never killed anyone: it will just make you a better public speaker next time.

If you can do this as you go through your routine and be more aware of your state of mind, then you'll find that you can prevent the stress response before it arises and rob your anxieties of all their power over you.

For more serious anxieties and phobias, you can even take this one step further and try what is known as 'hypothesis testing'. Here, you simply test your fears by standing up to them and letting them happen. For example, you would go out onto the stage and *purposefully* stutter. You'll find that no one laughs and nothing bad comes from it!

Conclusion

Hopefully at this point, you have all the tools and knowledge you need to begin reducing and combating the stress in your own life.

This isn't going to be an easy ride. Stress for many of us has become a normal part of life and habits are hard to change.

But by using meditation, you'll find that you can reduce your base level of stress and rebuild some of the damage to your brain caused by anxiety. What's more, is that this will teach you to be more aware of your thoughts and better able to control them and thereby steer your emotions.

It's time to wrestle back control of your mind. *You* tell your body when it needs to wake up and when it needs to focus. You decide what's worth worrying about. And when you're home and work is over, you use this power to allow yourself to rest, recover and forget all about the stresses of the day.

Once you can do all this, you'll find your mood improves, your productivity skyrockets and your health is greatly enhanced in both the long *and* short term.

Stress less, live more.